D1617128

Seven Keys to Surviving the Trump Presidency

Dr. Calm's Prescription for Healing Post-Election Stress

Kiran Dintyala, MD, MPH, ABIHM

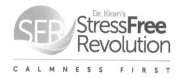

Dr. Kiran's
Stress**Free**
Revolution

CALMNESS FIRST

Printed in the United States of America

First Printing: January 2017

978-0-9986508-1-4 (paper)
978-0-9986508-2-1 (ebook)

Providence Press

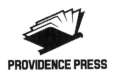

PROVIDENCE PRESS

Contents

About the Author

Dr. Kiran Dintyala is an internal medicine physician, practicing full time in Palm Springs, California. He is an author, speaker, and stress-management expert. He also holds a Master's in Public Health (MPH), and during his studies, he learned stress-management skills.

His mission is to elevate the emotional well-being of humanity and thus increase the happiness index of this world.

Every day, Dr. Dintyala compassionately takes steps to alleviate the suffering of humanity and empower people to succeed in their lives through better usage of their own innate capabilities to be happy, peaceful, and content.

He firmly believes that with the simple principles and techniques he teaches, anyone can become stress-free. He envisions and strives toward creating stress-free organizations, communities, and families across the United States and the rest of the world.

He proposes that a calm state of mind greatly enhances our

productivity and capabilities in life, thus paving a path for success and happiness. Some of the benefits of a calm mind are as follows:

- **Peaceful and joyful living**
- **Achieving work–life balance**
- **Ability to perform under pressure**
- **Positive relationships at work and home**
- **Relaxed & motivating work environment**
- **Creating time to achieve what matters most in life**
- **Transforming organizational state of mind**
- **Reduced absenteeism and presenteeism**
- **Meeting important deadlines**
- **Better financial performance**

A Short Version of My Story

Many years ago, when I was in the middle of a perfect storm of stress in my life, I accidentally stumbled upon certain principles and techniques that saved my life. Those principles and techniques helped me calm down instantaneously and gave me the ability to take control of my life situation. That ability to calm down in the midst of chaos not only saved me from a dismal failure that threatened my career but also paved a path to the career of my dreams. *The concepts I have learned over years of many life-and-death situations became solidified into the P-E-T system for stress-free living* (more on this later). This system is simple and easy to follow, and it melts away stress instantaneously. These principles and techniques work with mathematical accuracy!

Why am I doing this?

Why did I choose this journey to create a stress-free revolution? Having benefited from this system myself, I am now on a journey to help others reap the same benefits. I know stress is a relentless killer. I have experienced extremes of stress in my own life, and I know how it feels to be in a situation that makes you feel desperate, hopeless, and unhappy. When you are in deep distress, you feel as if nothing works in your life. You feel as if everything is wrong in your life. You feel that there is no meaning to life. All the goals and dreams of life look futile. *Yet, with experience, I realized that there is a golden path to peaceful, joyful, and productive living.* No situation is hopeless and that there are obvious ways to emerge out of difficult situations successfully and find solutions.

There is a Tremendous Need to Eliminate Stress from Our Lives

Stress is recognized as a global epidemic by the United Nations. Stress management is Corporate America's greatest challenge in the 21st century. Families are falling apart because of stress. Individuals are losing focus in their lives and rapidly moving toward failure and depression because of stress. Yet, there is not enough preparedness to fight stress in our current society. There are obvious ways to fight stress and live a peaceful and joyful life. I am here to be your guide and offer a helping hand so that you can be peaceful and joyful too.

Start Your Stress-Free Journey Today!

The concepts I teach are simple, yet powerful. You will be amazed by the tremendous positive impact they will have on your life, professionally and personally! You will learn ways to be happy at home and work. You will learn innovative techniques to transform your organization and your family in a positive way. You don't have to agree with me blindly. Experiment with these concepts. You will be pleasantly surprised by the magnitude of the positive results!

Acknowledgments

First and foremost, I am thankful to God and my Guru, Paramhansa Yogananda, for this life and their visible and invisible guidance at every step of my life, including the manifestation of this book.

I am deeply indebted to my parents and my sister for their steadfast love and support, without which I would not have developed into the person and the professional I am today.

My wife, Mariana, who believes in my knowledge and abilities, and who is my strongest advocate and staunchest critic. I am grateful for her love, friendship, and support.

Our daughter Mayura, who gives meaning to my life and without whom I can't live, inspires me every day to progress and prosper in life. In her beautiful ways, she reminds me to live life to the fullest every moment.

I am deeply grateful for the tremendous support provided by Martha Bullen, Geoffrey Berwind, Gail Snyder, Raia King, Nick Ippoliti, and Dave and Heidi Grauel. Without their dedication to this project, it wouldn't have been possible to publish this book.

Thanks to Dave Grauel for the eye catching design work and Heidi Grauel for her wonderful editorial work. Both of them worked diligently to make this book come to life even though they were in the midst of an unexpected crisis and had very busy schedules. I appreciate their dedication, integrity, and excellence.

Special thanks goes to Martha Bullen for her tremendous support and phenomenal advice on book writing, marketing, and publishing. Literally, she held my hand and helped me through each and every single step of the complex process of book writing and publishing. Without her sincere support it wouldn't have been possible for this book to see the light of this world.

I deeply appreciate Nick Ippoliti, my web designer, who has become my good friend, for his conscientious advice and marketing expertise for making this book the best possible success it can be.

I am also deeply indebted to my family, friends, and colleagues for their advice and support in my life—whenever I needed them, they were there.

Serenity Prayer

God,

Grant Me the Serenity

To Accept the Things, I Cannot Change,

Courage to Change the Things I can,

And

The Wisdom to Know the Difference.

Preface

Our nation is in great turmoil. The deep divide between liberals and conservatives is more evident now than ever. Daily I witness various people at work, home, schools, and other locations getting into arguments over the impending Trump presidency. Before the election, for more than a year, people felt great anxiety about the future of our nation. The presidential candidate selection process for the Republican and Democratic Parties left deep feelings of hurt and disdain for many, both for the candidates and their supporters. People felt that the candidate selection process was not fair, the media coverage was dishonest and biased, the journalists shunned their responsibility to report the truth, and dirty politics were given precedence over the true north principles on which this nation was founded.

By the time the final two presidential candidates for the Democratic and Republican Parties were selected, many were left in shock and felt unsettled. Many people felt that these candidates were unqualified and vastly different and that both lacked moral authority. Both candidates were deeply disliked by citizens of the United States. The undesirable ratings for both candidates were at historical highs. Yet, we had no choice but to accept the nominees. There was huge dissent (in both parties) regarding the character flaws, personalities, and murky histories of both candidates. The people of the nation, who were faced with the vital decision of choosing their future president from one of these less desirable candidates, wished they had a better choice. Alas! There was no other choice. Although the Green Party and the Libertarian Party candidates did run for the presidency, they never gained the traction needed to become viable alternatives.

So, we, the people, made up our mind to support the candidate who we felt would best lift our nation from its enormous debt of 20 trillion dollars, stimulate the economy, create more jobs, reduce taxes, improve healthcare for all, reduce the crime rate in our inner cities, stop the drug overflow over the border, dismantle the corrupt Washington politics, secure our nation from outside forces, defeat terrorism, and finally bring back the America we all want—a peaceful, prosperous, and powerful nation that is invincible to even the deadliest of its enemies, that is supportive of the needs of the nations that are its friends, and that is kind and generous to all the people of this world.

We, the people, have eagerly waited to be liberated from the shackles of mediocrity, revive our greatness, and realize our American dreams! So, the final day that would decide the fate of our nation had come, Election Day. The preceding few weeks before the election couldn't have been more stressful. Political commentators, pundits, long-time journalists, and experienced Washington insiders have pronounced that this election season was unprecedented in the history of America in its intensity, animosity, ill-will, and terribly negative political campaigning.

On the day of the election, November 8, 2016, I thought, as did many others, that all of this turmoil, commotion, and agitation would come to an end. Election Day had come; the results were out, and the president-elect was announced. With the election of our 45th president, many thought they could put their minds at rest, go back to their daily routines, and move on with their lives. People were hoping to heal their hearts, forget their differences, get along with others at work and home, and forgo all the negativity this election had brought upon them. However, as days passed, I noticed that was not the case. The election had resulted in a deeply divided nation.

Many in the nation felt extremely disgruntled by the election result and could not accept it. Many people could not come to terms with the reality of a Trump presidency. Social media had become a conduit to vent their deeply unhappy feelings. Riots broke out. People were shouted at, shot at, and hurt, among many other unfortunate events. There were protests both within and outside of Washington, DC.

I thought, "With all this negativity and divisiveness gripping the people, will our nation ever heal?" As I spoke casually with colleagues, friends, acquaintances, family, and clients, I saw that at least half of the nation couldn't see a way out of the stress they had been experiencing over the election cycle. Even months after, many still find it difficult to sleep peacefully at night. At work and home, these people feel fearful and anxious about their and their nation's future.

As a stress reduction expert, when I see people suffering every day, I can't help but ask myself, "How can I help them? What can I do to make them feel better? Wouldn't it be great if I could show them a way out of this deep distress?" I clearly see the solution for the stress that resulted from this election. It's possible to heal. It's possible to feel normal again. Peace of mind is attainable. I have put together some important tips on how to handle "election stress" and have shared it with people around me.

The response I received was overwhelming. People found these tips helpful and soothing to their souls. I had wanted to write a small book on this topic earlier but refrained from doing so because the election was already over and I thought people would soon forget about it. But even now, I still see a lot of agitation and anxiety over this issue. There is a lot of reluctance to accept the election results and move on. Celebrities, Hollywood stars, and politicians have openly expressed their dissent, which has stirred huge controversies. If this continues, it will be very hard for our nation to heal. So, I thought, writing a book that helps people get over the post-election stress is timely and will serve many. And here it is. I hope people find this book helpful in releasing stress and finding peace of mind.

Introduction
Post-Election Stress Disorder

The election has left millions of people in a state of great distress that they can't escape. I call this post-election stress disorder. What is post-election stress disorder? To know that, first we should define stress and understand the difference between acute stress and chronic stress.

Stress at its core is nothing but a state of mind in which you feel unhappy and distressed. Acute stress response is your body's physiological response to a stressful situation. Stressful situations can be an illness, a threat to life, or an event like an election. Once you feel distressed in your mind, your brain and body release stress hormones (like cortisol and adrenaline), which lead to stress symptoms and signs like palpitations, rapid heart rate, nausea, fainting, and chest pain, among others. Usually, this acute stress response dissipates in an hour or so. If it continues for days, weeks, or months, it is called chronic stress.

What turns an acutely stressful event into chronic stress? Repetitive, persistent thinking about the stressful event causes chronic stress. Often, these stressful events happen once, but people continue to think about them for a long time and perpetuate stress in their lives. Sometimes, the stressful event has not happened yet, but people imagine a fearful future and respond to it in a stressful way and make their lives miserable. For example, Donald Trump was elected as our president on November 8, 2016. Obviously, millions of Clinton supporters became extremely distressed as a result. That's understandable, and there is nothing wrong with that. If you supported Hillary Clinton, it is expected that you would be upset about the election result.

But, that's not the problem. *People are not just upset for a few hours or a few days, which is alright and very human. The problem is that people are living in that perpetual state of distress for months, and this situation may extend for years.* As of this writing, it has been more than two months since the election, and I see people who are more upset now compared with two months ago. People are chronically stressed about the election result. They continue to react to the event that is no longer present. They tend to imagine a fearful future under a Trump presidency, and they don't know how to handle it. I call this perpetual state of worry, anxiety, anger, fear, insecurity, and uncertainty after the election result, post-election stress disorder (PESD).
Post-election stress disorder is a real phenomenon that's happening in our nation right now. One of my psychiatry friends received 47 phone calls the night Donald Trump was elected. People were freaking out. This is not fiction; it is a real event that happened in real time.

Consider the following story.

One day, at 7:00 am in the morning, I got a call from the nurse that the blood pressure (BP) of one of my patients was uncontrollable. It was 200/110. Oh, my God! That's high. As many of you may already know, high BP can lead to stroke, heart attack, and other devastating health problems. "Let's give him some extra medications intravenously," I told the nurse. The patient was admitted to the hospital, and for the next two days, we tried various methods to control his BP, but it wouldn't come down easily. We had to almost double the number of medications he was taking before we finally got his BP controlled. I said to myself, "There must be a reason why his BP shot up so high. Let me see what's going on. Something must be going on here." So, I sat next to the patient and asked him, "Have you been taking all your BP meds at home?" He replied, "Yes, I have been taking them regularly. I don't miss a single pill." "Have you been taking a lot of salt in your diet?" I asked. "Not at all. In fact, I have cut down the amount of salt I take significantly over the past few months," he replied.

I was puzzled. *Noncompliance with diet and not taking medications are two common reasons for uncontrollable BP in patients with hypertension.* I thought to myself, "Then, what would have caused his BP to go up?" I asked him, "Tell me what's going on in your life. Have you been stressed lately?" And that made him open up! He immediately said, "You bet. I am so stressed! This Trump thing is killing me. Every time I watch TV, my BP shoots up sky high. I am so stressed about all this election stuff." Then I said, "The election is over. What's stressing you about it now?"

He replied, "Well, I want to get over it and come to terms and accept our new president, but our media won't let it go. As soon as you turn on the TV, they constantly discuss how to get rid of him, why he shouldn't be the president, how to overthrow him, and all the other negative stuff. As much as I want to let it go, the constant focus on this issue by media is making it hard for me to let it go." I laughed and said, "Why do you watch all that negative news? Why don't you watch something else on TV?"

He gave a big sigh and replied, "I know. I am trying. But, it's so hard not to be dragged into the media sensationalism. You are constantly bombarded with all this news, and it's hard to avoid it. If not TV, it's there in newspapers. If not newspaper, it's there on social media and our phones. My iPhone constantly sends me these stupid news reminders. I should disable it. I am going to try not to take in all this negative information. I know that's not good for me and my health."

At that point, I gave my patient some relaxation exercises and tips on how to get over election stress, and soon his BP came down. I cut his medications in half. That's the power of addressing the root cause of any problem. In this case, it was stress. Once my patient's stress levels decreased, there was no difficulty in decreasing his BP.

High BP is not the only way your body exhibits stress; your overall health can also deteriorate. *Stress is associated with the six leading causes of death in the United States: heart disease, cancer, lung disease, stroke, suicide, and accidents.* Stress leads to rapid aging. Stress makes you prone to addictions. Stress degrades your immune system and thus makes you susceptible to infections. Stress can trigger autoimmune diseases. Poor sleep due to stress can increase the risk of having seizures.

The devastating effects of stress do not stop there. Stress leads to poor relationships, both at work and home. Eventually, this can result in a divorce or a job loss or some other terrible consequence. Stressed people can become depressed and commit suicide. Low self-esteem and loss of self-confidence are other major symptoms in stressed people. Stressed people tend to make more mistakes and thus get themselves and others around them in trouble. The list of all the bad consequences of stress is endless. So, let's stop here and move on to find solutions to the stresses of life. *The solution to PESD is to disconnect the link between acute and chronic stress.* How do you do that? That's what this book is here to tell you. Read on.

Key No. 1
Prioritize Peace of Mind

Peace of Mind Matters

The first step in finding the solution to the stress resulting from the election (PESD) is to acknowledge the fact that your peace of mind is more important than anything else. Only if you have peace of mind, do all the money, possessions, and power you have in life matter. If you lack it, then all the money and power in the world can't make you happy. So, don't lose your peace of mind for anything. *Do whatever you have to do without losing peace of mind. That's the essence of the art of stress-free living.*

The reason I emphasize this point so strongly is that I often see people throwing away their peace of mind like a piece of garbage that has no value (and for reasons that are quite regretful). *The very concept of peace of mind is not given enough importance in our culture.* People place a lot of value in money, relationships, possessions (such as cars, homes, phones, and computers), and political power, but rarely is peace of mind seen as an entity that needs to be valued and retained by all means. That concept doesn't exist in our modern society. Thus, people get into petty arguments in their relationships, giving more importance to ego than to peace to mind. People trade in their mental peace in the pursuit of making more money. People jeopardize their peace of mind in the struggle to amass political power and climb higher and higher up the ladder in their organization.

Most People Lack Peace of Mind Because It's Not a Priority for Them

The result is, obviously, that most people lack peace of mind and are deeply stressed. The truth is you can't solve the problem of stress unless you prioritize peace of mind. So, make up your mind now that you are going to do whatever it takes to regain your peaceful self. The reason this is so important is that when someone is peaceful, he or she tends to be more energetic and healthier, be more helpful and kinder to others, perform better at work, make better decisions in life, and much more. *Overall, a person lives a much more harmonious and wholesome life when he or she is peaceful.* And who doesn't want that? We all do. And that is what this book is about.

Being Busy Is Not an Excuse to Throw Away Your Peace of Mind

Let me give you an example that demonstrates this point. Recently, I had been very busy doing multiple projects, including writing a book, creating a video program on stress management, performing stress management research, dealing with some problems with the home I was living in, handling an unexpected situation where one of my close relatives was diagnosed with cancer, attending a few back-to-back conferences, and so on. All this was happening on top of a very hectic schedule as a physician. Initially, I was very happy that all the stress management work that I wanted to do was going so well. But eventually, all these different priorities started encroaching into the calm space within and eating away my peace of mind as I kept missing my "quiet time," which, for me, is meditation that I regularly do.

As I continued to engage myself in these other activities, I started to feel very restless. Things were not flowing well. I felt very low in energy and became easily tired. At one point, it started impacting my health. I lost my appetite. Whatever I ate didn't taste right and wasn't being digested easily. I felt palpitations. The goals I set to achieve were not happening.

It Doesn't Take Much Time to Regain Your Peace of Mind

Finally, one day, I stopped myself and asked, "What's going on? Why don't I feel happy? Why don't I feel good that I am busy with the work I wanted to do? Is that not what I wanted? Why am I feeling so restless?" As I reflected upon this, I realized that I was ignoring my peace of mind and was doing everything else at its expense. I had de-prioritized my peace of mind. I realized my mistake. Immediately, I changed my priorities. I started doing yoga and meditation again, and immediately my energy came back. I felt vibrant, healthy, and, most importantly, peaceful. Things started flowing well in life again. My appetite was back, and I started eating well. I got back to the rhythm of being myself as soon as I prioritized peace of mind.

Do you know how long it took for me to get back into the groove? Just one day. Yes, all it took was one day! *The moment I prioritized peace of mind and took actions to promote it, I started feeling better. That's a huge point!* All you need to do to feel well and de-stress is to prioritize your peace of mind and take the necessary actions to make it happen. By choosing to read this book, you have already taken a step toward achieving peace of mind. Read on.

 Dr. Calm's Recommended Exercises

1. For the next week, no matter what happens, be determined to remain peaceful.

2. When a negative news attracts your attention, stop for a moment and ask yourself if it is worth losing your peace of mind for this.

3. If a family member, friend, or colleague makes a comment you don't like, ask yourself whether that's worth arguing and getting into a fight.

4. When protesters rally against our president, ask yourself if that's going to help do good for anyone or if it is a selfish act.

5. Allot yourself not more than 15 minutes a day for you to be up-to-date on the news. That's ample time to learn the major news events of the day without getting dragged into instigating details.

6. If possible, for the next three weekends, go away somewhere you won't be bothered by anyone and where you can relax and regain your peace of mind.

7. Make sure you prioritize your peace of mind. Keep your quiet time appointment as if you would keep the appointment with the most important person of your dreams.

Key No. 2
Acceptance

When the Whole World Got It Wrong

Coming to terms with the election result and accepting Donald Trump as president are difficult for many people, especially liberals. If you are a liberal, you probably had written off Trump long ago. When Trump got nominated by the Republican Party, most Democrats thought that the race was over and that Hillary Clinton was sure to become the next President of the United States. When the "locker room" video of Mr. Trump emerged in early October, most people, including conservatives, thought that was the end of Donald Trump. All the polls declared that Mr. Trump would never win. *Everyone was just waiting for Election Day just to complete the formality of electing Mrs. Clinton as our future president.*

So, on the night of November 8, when one state after another started turning red, most people were a little surprised. But still, they thought it was impossible for Mr. Trump to win without overturning at least a couple of blue states. So, liberals were comfortable and conservatives still wary for a while that evening. However, as the early votes from Wisconsin and Michigan started coming in, Mrs. Clinton's supporters started feeling uneasy. Trump supporters were happy but were still not sure of a victory. *I was stuck to the TV like millions of other people across the nation and around the world, eagerly waiting for the final results.*

When Trump Won

The political analysts on CNN, Fox, NBC, and other major news media outlets were rapidly analyzing the electoral college votes state by state, reshuffling the votes per the latest results, and they started seeing that *a path to victory for Donald Trump was not only plausible but also quite close to possible.* Still, even with the feeling of unease and racing hearts, liberals were hoping that the early results from Michigan and Wisconsin would revert and propel Clinton back to lead in those deep blue states. Meanwhile, initially, Pennsylvania looked good for Democrats and did not even seem to be on the table for Republicans.

So, Republicans were hoping that Trump would win Michigan and Wisconsin and that if he won New Hampshire, then he would have a chance to win the election. However, events unfolded in a very different way than expected, shocking almost everyone in the United States. The initial sizeable lead that Mrs. Clinton had maintained in *the Democratic firewall state of Pennsylvania started cracking down*, and Mr. Trump slowly but steadily gained on her, closing the gap and opening a massive lead as the votes from rural counties across Pennsylvania started coming in. People watched this phenomenon incredulously and couldn't believe what they were seeing. I, personally, started changing channels from one to another just to make sure what I was seeing was not an error in reporting.

The faces of the people at the Democratic election night party at Javits Center in New York City reflected deep shock and disbelief. What was supposed to be an easy win and a celebratory time was suddenly turned into a ghostly night with the terrible news etched deeply into their minds. *It was as if the beautiful dream-like feeling they were experiencing was suddenly replaced with the worst nightmare of their life—the thing that they most feared and least expected.* Around midnight in New York, the final results had not yet been announced. All liberals and Democrats were hoping for a miracle to turn the results upside down, but that miracle never happened.

The Trillion-Dollar Question

Shortly after midnight, in the early hours of November 9th, Mrs. Clinton conceded defeat in a private call to Mr. Trump. *Many around the world watched with dismay, appalled at this completely unexpected and totally impossible phenomenon—the Trump Phenomenon.* How was it possible for him to win? Almost everyone, including his own party, had written him off from the election books for a long time. Almost the whole world was against him, including the Democrats, the media, the political elites and pundits on both sides of the aisle, and even some Republicans.

How was it possible for Trump to win? This is the trillion-dollar question that has plagued almost every liberal in the country. His unfavorable ratings were at an all-time high, his likeability was at a historical low, and the negative ads and attacks against him were viciously powerful. How was it possible? How did this man endure all this and still manage to win?

When people talk about the difficulty in moving on and accepting the election results, all these events and thoughts come to their mind, making it difficult for them to move on. The experiences of this election cycle have left many bereft of peace of mind. Many have developed severe anxiety. Many feel as though the thing they feared the most has come true and they do not know how to adjust to this new reality. *Many are genuinely concerned about the future of their country, just as they are concerned about the future of their own families and themselves.* So, for these people, it is hard to move on. And this is perfectly understandable. I can put myself in their shoes and feel their pain. Thus, I have decided to do something that could help them relieve their stress, regardless of their faith or partisanship, whether they are liberal, a disgruntled conservative, or an independent.

There Is No Point in Continuing the Resentment

Now that the election is over, we must ask a question. Is there a point in continuing to resist the idea of a Trump presidency? Would reluctance help you to move forward in life and have a bright future? *Is it worth thinking about the absurdity of all this over and over again and worrying about it? Is it worth throwing away your peace of mind and suffering for the next four years, constantly reminding yourself of the horror from the election night?* I personally think it's not worth it. But, no one can answer that question for you. Only you can answer it for yourself. The stress that results from this post-election stress disorder (PESD) can be harmful to your health, peace, and prosperity! Then why perpetuate it? Let's decide today to put an end to it. But how? That's another trillion-dollar question, and this time, fortunately, I think I have the answer.

There Is a Plan . . . a Universal Plan

The first step is to realize that everything happens for a reason. *Even the worst possible events of your life happen for a reason.* You may not see the reason now, but eventually, it will be evident to you. There is no greater truth than this. Events have happened in my life that caused great pain and suffering, and I used to think, "Is this really necessary? Why do I have to go through this? What's the purpose of all this suffering?" Often, I used to have no answers at that time, but months or even years later, the answer would emerge, and it would be very evident why certain events happened in my life. Meanwhile, I became stronger. Those events changed the direction of my life for the better, and without those events, I would have never changed. So, be patient, have faith, and eventually, the right time will come for you to know the answers.

All Failures Are Not Bad

Let me give you a short example that demonstrates this point. A few years ago, one of my good friends came to me and offered a great investment opportunity. He said that not many people knew about it, but because he was an insider at a certain investment company he knew it would be a great opportunity and he immediately invested a lot of money and wanted me to do the same. I was naturally excited, and after considering the details of the investment, I found it to be a great opportunity and decided to go ahead and invest in it. It required a lot of money, close to $100,000, but I didn't have that amount of money available at the time. I tried to gather what I could, but it was not sufficient. I struggled for a few months, but my efforts didn't come to fruition. I felt bad that I had lost a golden opportunity.

Sometimes It's Better Not to Succeed

Well, what could I do except move on and forget about the investment? So, I did. I thought maybe there was a reason why it didn't happen although I couldn't see the reason at the time. It was a low-risk investment with good returns; so what could go wrong? Two years later, I suddenly remembered the investment and decided to inquire about it. I called my friend and asked how it was going. He said, "Well, this did not go well. Initially it took off well, but later it all became very chaotic. There is a lawsuit going on now, and there is nothing wrong from our side, but there are people involved in this deal that are not so nice. Overall, it's complicated and I don't know what's going to happen." I felt bad for him, but at the same time, I was relieved because I would have been in deep financial trouble had I invested in this opportunity with borrowed money.

There Is Always a Reason

You see, there was a reason why I didn't succeed in grabbing this so-called golden opportunity that turned out to be a disaster. I would have never expected this kind of outcome given the facts I knew at the outset. In the end, I was saved from a lot of trouble because I did not get what I wanted—the investment opportunity. There is always a reason. Many such events have happened in my life, and *I no longer doubt the judgment of the Almighty regarding the way things are carried out in this world.* There is always a reason. I am sure Mr. Trump has become our next president for a reason as well. We will all find that out soon.

One last thing to remember is that life is not perfect. You don't always get what you want. That's the harsh truth of life. Once you accept this fact, life becomes more enjoyable. Read on.

 Dr. Calm's Recommended Exercises

1. When feelings of resistance to Trump's presidency come to your mind, ask yourself, "Is it worth to continue the resentment? Is that going to help maintain my peace of mind?" If it doesn't, let go of the resistance and be at peace with yourself.

2. Ask yourself, "How would I feel if half the people at my workplace and complete strangers resented me and did

not accept me?" What would be your reaction? Would
you like it?

3. Think, "Is Mr. Trump reacting to all the negative
incoming from the liberals, people in White House,
media, protesters, and much more?" How would you
react if almost everyone were against you? Would you
justify your actions? Is that what Mr. Trump is doing?

4. Ask yourself, "If I am accepted as I am, does that
make me feel less threatened or more rebellious?" Are
you ready to give that acceptance to Mr. Trump and
others? Do you think that will help Mr. Trump to be less
rebellious against his adversaries?

5. Do you believe in God's justice? Were you ever given
chances to correct your mistakes? Where you ever given
forgiveness? Isn't it healing? Don't you want to let our
nation heal through your acceptance?

6. Ask yourself at least once a day, "Who am I to judge?
Do I really know all the necessary details to make a
judgment? Don't we just have fragmented information
projected by media for the most part?" Most
information we get is not firsthand info. There are many
layers through which the information goes through
before it comes to us, the people. Then how can we make
an accurate judgment without accurate information?

Key No. 3
Arise, Awaken, and March Forward

Failure Is the Stepping Stone for Success

If you look at the history of this world, it becomes quite evident that successful people are not the ones who never failed but are those who did not let the failures deter them from their righteous goal. *It is not how many times you fall that matters but how many times you get up and march forward.* So, get up every time you fall. Never be discouraged and disheartened. Never lose hope. You fought well and did the best you could to help Hillary win, but sometimes, even after you give your best, things may not happen the way you want. There is nothing you can do but accept it and move forward.

Realize that failure is the stepping stone for success. Ask yourself what you can learn from the experience. What can you do better next time when faced with a similar situation? Do not dwell on negative feelings. *Do not self-criticize. Just self-evaluate, learn, and move on.* Of course, it is easier said than done. So, I am going to share with you the two natural gifts you have hidden within you. Those gifts are innate health and resiliency. We are born with these gifts.

Being Happy and Peaceful Is Natural to Us

Innate health is your natural state of mind where your happiness is unconditional and your peace of mind is independent of external circumstances. It means peace and joy are your true nature and innate qualities. This means *you don't have to depend on election results to determine your happiness or sadness.* Does this sound strange? It may initially because no one has ever told you this truth before. However, the more you understand this truth, the more evident it will be in your life.

Let me share with you an example that makes it easier to understand this. Have you ever watched children? They are so naturally happy, right? They often are at peace with themselves, right? We have an 18-month-old daughter, and she brings so much joy into our lives. Yes, occasionally she cries and wants this toy or that toy, but her distress over anything doesn't last any longer than a few minutes. The other day, she wanted to play with a fork, but we didn't give it to her because it's a pointed object and she could hurt herself with it. She became upset and started crying, but she soon turned her attention to something else and started playing again.

See, her happiness is not dependent on external circumstances. She is innately happy and peaceful. Once in a while, she feels like she wants a toy or some other object, but she knows that toy doesn't equate with her happiness, so it doesn't bother her when the toy is broken or lost. Looking at children, we can quickly learn that peace of mind and happiness are our true nature.

You don't have to achieve anything external to feel happy and peaceful. An illusion that millions of us continue to believe is that happiness can only be found by achieving some goal, making more money, being in power, or having more possessions. Again, this is an illusion. *Your happiness and peace of mind always lie within. That's the truth. Only to the extent you forget this truth will you feel unhappy.*

Do Not Equate Happiness with Your Circumstances

This doesn't mean that you should not make money, buy things, be in power, or achieve your goals. It's okay to do all those things, but don't equate your happiness with them. *The more you identify your happiness with those external conditions, the harder it will be for you to stay happy* when those external conditions are challenged. In this case, your desire for Mrs. Clinton to win was thwarted, and that brought upon you great distress. In addition, it's the dislike or hatred for Trump that is making you feel unhappy. Your dependence on these external circumstances is the root cause for your stress.

But remember that once upon a time you were perfectly happy without either of these conditions. You were born naturally happy. Just remember that, and you can get back to that state of unconditional happiness. But how do you get back there?

You Can Bounce Back Even
from the Most Difficult Situations

Your second divine gift, your inner resilience, helps you bounce back from a stressful state of mind to a peaceful state of mind. *Resilience is your inborn capacity to face the challenges of life with grace and to be flexible in life situations.* It is your capacity to stay strong in the midst of difficult circumstances. It's your capacity to reclaim your lost peace and joy in life. The power of human resilience winning against the odds of life's greatest vicissitudes has been demonstrated again and again throughout history. Many inspiring men and women have stood as examples of the indestructible nature of human resilience.

Let me share with you a real-life story that demonstrates the power of resilience. Recently, I was taking care of a patient who came in with a loss of appetite, significant weight loss, and some fluid accumulation in his belly. We did some tests, and as suspected, they came back positive for advanced cancer. I went in to deliver this news to him. When he heard the news, he said, "Okay, cool. What do we do next?"

I thought that I must have heard him wrong and was looking at him incredulously. He saw the expression on my face and said, "Yes, I did say cool! That sounds crazy, right? But, what do I do? Do you want me to worry because of the diagnosis I received? Is it going to change anything? Is it going to revert my diagnosis? No, right? So, I would rather take this news positively and move on. I have confidence that my body can heal. Let's see what happens. I am not worried about it."

The Indomitable Nature of the Human Spirit

That's an amazing story of someone who demonstrated the power of resilience under trying circumstances. He is also a powerful example of someone who did not abandon his innately peaceful nature as a result of an external event, in this case, a cancer diagnosis. If a person who has an advanced life-threatening cancer can defy stress and remain peaceful, I am sure we can do the same while facing the Trump presidency. My point is that *you have the ability to bounce back to your normal self and feel peaceful again despite the election result.*

Watch Life with Curiosity as It Unfolds

Many presidents have come and gone. Many natural disasters have come and gone. Many terrible things have happened in the history of the world. And still we survived, right? Life goes on, and all events of life will fade away with time. Why worry and lose your happiness over the Trump presidency? This too shall pass. It's just a matter of time. It's better to accept the result and be at peace than being in constant consternation over it. Be patient; be an innocent bystander and watch what's going to unfold with curiosity but not with animosity. With this attitude, you will be sure to find peace of mind.

You may ask: Do I have these divine gifts within me, or are they possessed by only a fortunate few? The answer is that yes you do have these gifts. These divine gifts are not a privilege bestowed upon select people based on race, color, money, social status, national origin, or any other external characteristic. *We are all born with the gifts of innate health and resilience.* They are just waiting for you to tap into them. Just awaken, arise, and march forward, and you will find that these gifts will shower peace of mind onto you. How do we tap into these gifts? Read on.

 Dr. Calm's Recommended Exercises

1. Once a week, take at least a few minutes to spend time in nature. It could be a park, it could be a beach, or it could be as simple as looking into the sky and enjoying the peace that is inherent in nature. Know that you are an inherent part of the nature and so your nature is peace, too. Feel it. Be it.

2. Close your eyes and imagine that you are relaxing next to an ocean. Feel the sound of the waves gently caressing the shore every few minutes. See that the waves are ever-changing and tumultuous. But, also recognize that the ocean beneath those waves is steadily peaceful and restful. Such is your true nature. The events in your life are like those superficial waves. Your true nature is peaceful like the ocean beneath. Remind yourself of this at least once a day.

3. This week, decide to do any new activity, an activity that you have never done before. It could be something

like playing tennis or as simple as buttoning your shirt with your non-dominant hand. When you do this activity, notice how difficult it is for you to do. But, also notice as you continue to do it every day, it becomes easier. The same way the more you use your power of resilience, the easier it becomes for you to be resilient and be strong during difficult circumstances. Remind yourself of your resilient nature every day.

Key No. 4
Practice Presence

Do Not Get Caught Up in the Past or the Future

Most people are stressed because they step out of the present moment and their minds get caught up thinking about the past or the future. Take, for example, the election. The results were out on November 9th, which was months ago. However, most people are still feeling the effects of the election—anxiety, anger, fear, worry, frustration, depression, altercations, and more. All these effects are the symptoms of post-election stress disorder (PESD). Why are these effects still being felt? Isn't it true that an acute stress response should dissipate in a few hours at most?

Let's take a closer look at this. Acute stress response is a normal physiological response of your body to an acutely stressful event. Let me give you an example. If a zebra is being hunted down by a lion, the acute stress response, which is a fight-or-flight response, helps it escape from the lion, and once it escapes, the acute stress response dissipates in an hour or so. The zebra returns to its normal state, grazes, mixes with the herd, and moves on. Do you see how the Zebra is not holding onto the stressful event? If the same thing happens to you, a human being, what do you think happens?

The Story of a Lion and the Human

First, hopefully you escape. It's not going to be an easy task as the fastest human being can only sprint at 20 miles per hour and an average lion can easily outrun you at 45 miles per hour. However, let's say a miracle happened and you escaped. You ran back to the bus you came from on the African safari tour, and you sit there for a while in shock. Once you recover, you think, "Why did this lion attack me? What's wrong with it? I am a good person. This lion has no business to attack me. I paid for this safari tour. I am not trespassing. And why me? There are a hundred other people here. Why did the lion attack me? I am an animal lover. I have five dogs and 10 cats at home, and I take care of them well. The lion should know this. This is inappropriate. I will report this lion to the tour officials. . . " And your mind goes on and on and on.

Now, you tell the story to the fellow passengers in the bus all day. Then you go back to your hotel, and that night, you can't sleep well because you keep waking up with nightmares. The next day, you call your friends and family who are thousands of miles away and narrate the story again and curse the lion. After you finish the African safari tour, you go home, and three months later, you still keep waking up in the middle of the night screaming, "Lion! Lion! Help me! Help me!" Well, now you have just been diagnosed with post-traumatic stress disorder (PTSD). The post-election stress disorder (PESD) is not much different from this.

The Root Cause of Chronic Stress

Do you see from this example how acute stress turned into chronic stress? Do you see how you continued to respond to an acute event that was no longer present? Do you know what led to chronic stress in this case? It was your thinking. More specifically, it was your ability as a human to misuse your thinking that resulted in chronic stress. To be stressed after the lion attacked you is a normal stress response. But to continue to stress about it for hours, days, weeks, and sometimes months is abnormal because you are continuing to respond to an event that's no longer present. The lion has long forgotten you, but you haven't forgotten the lion. That's the cause of all the chronic stress you have been experiencing.

Chronic stress results from dysfunctional, repetitive thinking about events that are not current. They can be events of the past or future events that haven't happened yet. Either way, we use our power of thinking against ourselves, either by ruminating on the past or by imagining a fearful future, and bring stress upon ourselves. This is the root cause of all chronic stress in our lives.

Your Inquiry into the Future Can Be Endless; Do Not Fall into That Trap

With regard to the election, when Mr. Trump won, millions of people around the world were expectedly shocked. That's an acute stress response. But the condition of people repeatedly continuing to react to the election weeks and months later is what is turning that acute stress into chronic stress. People are not only reacting to what happened but are also imagining a very dire future and are extremely worried about it. What's going to happen to my country? What's going to happen to my job, family, and children? What's going to happen to our healthcare? Are we going to conflict with other nations about trade? Are we going to get into war with other countries? Is there going to be a nuclear war?

There is no end to the number of questions your mind can ask. However, has anything like that happened yet? Not yet, right? Then why stress about it? If worrying about things made them better, we should all worry together. But worrying does not make things any better. *Even if your worst fears come true, worrying and getting upset are not going to do you or others any good.* What you will reap, though, if you continue to stress is bad health. All the chronic stress accumulated in your life will lead to chronic disease. As I mentioned earlier, chronic stress is associated with the six leading causes of death. Most chronic diseases have their foundation in chronic stress. So, no matter how you look at it, there is no point in stressing about a situation.

Past and Future Don't Exist Anywhere Else Except Your Mind

Remember, *the past is nothing but a memory in your mind.* It's over. It no longer exists. All that exists is your thoughts about the past. The past has no life of itself other than what you breathe into it. And every one of us remembers the past in a different way. So, the reality you want to give to the past is entirely up to you. Either you can learn from it and move on, or you can continue to ruminate over it and make your life miserable.

Similarly, the future is nothing but a figment of your imagination. It is not here yet. It just exists in your mind because of your ability to think and project thoughts into the future. It has no life of itself. You create it. What kind of future do you want to create? A horrible one or a beautiful one? It's entirely up to you. Don't cling on to negative thoughts, lest you may create bad future. Hold on to good and positive thoughts and create a wonderful future.

Be Present

Anchor yourself to the present moment. The present moment is where everything happens. *Even the thoughts about the past and the future must be thought in the present. There is no other moment in life than the present moment.* Whatever happened a minute ago is already past. It just exists as a memory in your mind. Whatever is about to happen a minute from now is not here. It's just your imagination. There is only one moment—this moment. Enjoy every moment today because you can't predict what's going to happen tomorrow.

Let's say you will be driving to work tomorrow. You may get a flat tire, you may see an accident on the street that delays you, or you may have a smooth ride with no problems. But you don't know for sure exactly what's going to happen. *If you can't predict what's going to happen tomorrow in your own life, then how can you predict what's going to happen in politics and regarding national issues.* If you are like me, an average American, you don't have much say in any of those national issues. You have already cast your vote, and the election is over. So, forget about it. Get to work. Get back to your routine. Move on and march forward.

Your Destiny Is in Your Hands

Remember, in the end, *your destiny depends more on the conscious choices you make every day in your life than on the sporadic events like the election that happens every four years.* You have no control over what our president is going to do, but you do have control over what you can do in your life. That doesn't mean that our presidents do not alter the course of the nation. They do. However, remember that millions of people voted for previous presidents. If that were supposed to alter our lives dramatically, then by now all of us would be very happy and very rich. That didn't happen, right? At the end of the day, your destiny depends on your own actions. Your actions depend on your thoughts, your thoughts depend on your state of mind, and your state of mind depends on certain important factors that I am going to share with you in the next chapter. Read on.

Dr. Calm's Recommended Exercises

1. Take a moment every day in the morning when you wake up and ask yourself, "What is this moment? Present, past, or future?" Obviously, this is present. Then ask yourself, "Where are my thoughts? In the present or am I thinking about the past or future?" This simple exercise, if done once or twice a day, will transform your life. It will root you in the present.

2. Keep your eyes closed, observe your thoughts as they come and go. See how long each thought stays in your mind. Is it just for a moment or two that it lingers, after which the thought dissipates itself into nothingness? As you watch this closely, you become more and more present. As do you it longer, you connect more deeply with the present.

Key No. 5
Practice Calmness

Your State of Mind Determines the Quality of Your Thoughts and Vice Versa

If you are in a good state of mind, you are naturally going to have positive and happy thoughts, but bad thoughts will reign if you're in a poor state of mind. *Your mood and your thoughts are inseparably related to each other.* The whole field of stress management and prevention revolves around putting yourself in a good state of mind. But how do you do this? And how do you do it consistently?

My Story

To answer these questions, I will share with you a small but profound real-life story. Many years ago, when I was in deep distress because of a terrible event that happened in my life, I was enveloped by a vortex of negative thoughts. I had lost even the last ray of hope. Then, I accidentally stumbled upon certain principles and techniques that helped me calm down instantaneously. They helped me regain control over my mind and thus my life, and I went on to pursue a bright career and good life. At the time, I realized how powerful these principles and techniques are and how fortunate I was to stumble upon them.

Over the next few years, I noticed that friends, family, colleagues, and lot of other people were stressed and struggling to battle the challenges of life. I thought, "If only they knew these principles and techniques, they would not suffer so much." So, I decided to spread the message for the benefit of all. I have distilled the essence of all my study, research, insights, and experience into a breakthrough system called **The P-E-T System for Stress-Free Living**™.

It's designed to instill calmness, reduce stress, and improve the quality of life as a whole. A lot of good things have happened since I developed this system. Many people have benefited from this system, and I will share some of that information with you in this book. The description of the complete system is beyond the scope of this book. However, I will share with you its essence and the core concepts around which the system was built.

Calmness Is Your True Nature

First and foremost, a calm state of mind is your true nature. Although we all are born with it, most of us have drifted far from this calm state of mind and are stuck in a state of restlessness.

However, we can always bounce back to that calm state very quickly. *Your calmness is always just one step away. How do you reclaim it?*

Here are the three Laws of Thought Mechanics™ that help you reclaim your calmness and live a stress-free life.

The Laws of Thought Mechanics

1. **Thoughts flow freely in your mind, like water flows in the river. As long as thoughts flow freely in your mind, you remain in a naturally peaceful state of mind.**

2. **Stagnation of thoughts leads to stress. Stagnation results from attachment to thoughts.**

3. **Whatever thoughts you focus on becomes your reality. You create your reality through your own thoughts.**

Now, let's apply these laws to the current situation and see how they work. When the election results were announced and Mr. Trump emerged as the victor, many people became worried and afraid because they were thinking about how terrible Mr. Trump is, how bad the news was, how disappointed they were, and on and on. By keeping their focus on this negative information and becoming attached to negative thoughts in their minds, they created thought stagnation. That results in stress.

When the flow of water in a river is blocked, it leads to stagnation and thus the growth of bacteria and bugs, making the water unhealthy to drink. Something similar occurs when the flow of thoughts is blocked in your mind; it leads to thought stagnation and is unhealthy for your mind. Soon stress starts accumulating. People perpetuate the stress by continuing to think about the event, arguing about it with others, sharing their fears with others, and doing everything possible to detest Mr. Trump. Then they wonder why they are feeling stressed. People are stressed because they feel whatever they focus on. The more they focus on negative information, the worse they are going to feel.

The only solution is to let go of the negativity and focus on something positive. Focus on something you like. Just let go of all the resentment and anger. As Mark Twain remarked, "*Anger is an acid that can do more harm to the vessel in which it is stored than to anything on which it is poured.*"

So, enjoy life. Enjoy every moment. Forego all judgment. Who are we to judge? The ultimate judge, God Almighty, has been watching over everything. Be patient. Remember, there are no accidents. Everything happens in this universe for a reason. When you accept this truth, a great peace will dawn upon you.

Relaxation Exercise

Another thing you can do to find calm is to practice the relaxation exercise below. It helps a lot.

1. Lie down or sit back in an easy chair, and completely relax both your mind and body. Just let go of everything—every thought, idea, limitation, pain, every past event or future worry, every feeling, just

about everything that could possibly arise in your mind—and just relax completely and ease into your body and mind.

2. Breathe deeply and release your breath slowly. Again, breathe deeply and release slowly. Do it a few times, possibly for the next 2 to 3 minutes. You will feel your body and mind relaxing. Don't think about it, though. Just ease into your breathing.

3. Let your breathing take a natural rhythm and follow it. Your breathing will slow down and become very enjoyable and relaxing. Ease into it. Let it be. Let nothing bother you at this time. You are alone. You are free. You are enjoying yourself.

4. As you relax and ease into this state, you will feel all the restlessness in your body and mind completely dissolve. If you still feel a bit of restlessness, continue to ease into your breathing. Just let it be. If you want to, observe your breathing as it naturally happens.

5. Doing this exercise for 5 to 10 minutes is usually sufficient to completely relax you, but if you feel like you need to do it longer, that's fine, too. But within the first 5 minutes, you may notice yourself falling into a sleep-like state where you are deeply relaxed.

6. Rest there as long as you feel like before you return to your normal self. You will wake up feeling refreshed

and rejuvenated. Now your mind is clear, and you can carry on with your life and daily activities.

Meditation

Practicing meditation regularly helps a lot too. Choose any form of meditation you like, and I am sure you will benefit from it. The key to success in meditation is regularity. No matter how busy you are, don't miss your daily meditations. Before I elaborate on meditation, let me dispel any wrong beliefs about it.

What is meditation? Meditation is a state of mind in which you feel completely calm, where there is not even a flicker of restless thought in your mind. Until you reach that state, you are not really meditating. You are just practicing the technique, hoping to reach that meditative state. You may ask, "How do I know if have reached that state?"

My answer is that when you are there, you will know. You will feel a deep sense of peace and joy and a sense of deep security. You will feel that nothing can really bother you. To reach that state, however, you need to practice meditation daily and sincerely. Some people attain a meditative state of mind the first time they practice the technique. For others, it may take a little longer. With sincere effort and right technique, you will reach that state faster.

There are many techniques one can use to reach the state of meditation, and I will share with you one powerful technique below:

1. Sit upright in a chair or on the floor. Keep your spine erect and chin parallel to the ground. Avoid leaning your back against anything if possible.

2. Keep your mind and body relaxed. You could practice the relaxation exercise described earlier to relax your mind and body before practicing this technique. Let go of any tension in your body.

3. Close your eyes and look at the space between your two eyebrows. That's the location of your spiritual eye or third eye. There is no need to squint your eyes to look at the spiritual eye. Simply focus your attention there. If your eyes are restless and unfocused, don't be discouraged. Every time your gaze drifts away from the spiritual eye, bring it back gently to focus. With practice, you will be able to do so with ease.

4. Keeping attention on your spiritual eye, chant "peace" or "aum." Keep looking into the spiritual eye. Keep chanting internally. Get completely absorbed in the word you are chanting while you keep your gaze focused intently on the spiritual eye. The longer you do it, the easier it becomes.

5. If thoughts disturb you, ignore them. Know that all thoughts are transient. They just come and go. If you don't focus on them, they will go away. As you continue to do this, all your restless thoughts will subside, and at some point, you will suddenly feel a

deep sense of peace and joy. You will know it when
you feel it. When you feel it, stay with it. Don't inquire.
Don't think. Just stay with that feeling. Stay there as
long as possible.

6. You can do this technique as long as you want. I
suggest at least 20 minutes of practice a day and
longer if possible. As you start reaping the benefits of
meditation, you will automatically look forward to
your meditation time and will want to do it more and
more.

When you understand the laws of thought mechanics, practice
the relaxation exercise, and meditate regularly, a newfound grace
will bless your life, and you will be able to remain calm at will. As
you become calmer and calmer, you will find greater and greater
happiness in life. Things around you stop bothering you. You
will learn to take good and bad news equally. In other words,
you become even-minded, and this is the topic we are going to
explore in the next chapter—even-mindedness. Read on.

 Dr. Calm's Recommended Exercises

1. Remember, a calm state of mind is a good state of
mind and, in that state, the thoughts that arise in your
mind are positive and prosperous.

2. Be determined to remain calm no matter what. Even if people around you are restless, even when your surroundings are chaotic and when everyone is stressed out, you can remain calm, and you lead by example on how to remain calm.

3. The next time you are faced with a stressful situation, remember the Laws of Thought Mechanics. See what thoughts are bothering you. Then notice that your attachment to those thoughts is creating a stagnation in your mind, which is causing you stress. Then gently chose to move on and focus on something else that takes away your attention from negative thoughts.

4. At work or even at home, especially when you are stressed, take the time to practice the relaxation exercise. It helps de-stress. Take 5 minutes during lunch and do the exercise for your mid-day relaxation. Repeat the same at night for emptying your mind before sleep.

5. Never miss your daily meditations. If possible, do it the first thing in the morning, after taking a shower. If evenings are better for you, that's alright. Whatever time you decide on, do it every day the same time, if possible. That enhances the benefits you reap.

Key No. 6
Practice Even-Mindedness

The Nature of Life

Life is brutal. As soon as you think you vanquished one problem, another appears out of nowhere. That's the nature of life. It's full of surprises, some are good but some are really bad. How do you learn to remain unruffled when you are hit with bad news? How do you remain composed in the midst of challenges? How do you act with grace when your emotional fibers are stretched? To achieve that, you need to practice even-mindedness. What is even-mindedness? *Even-mindedness is the ability to remain neutral to all news, good and bad.* That doesn't mean that you don't get excited and feel happy when you receive good news. It just means that you don't get overly excited about it. You remind yourself that whatever good that you are experiencing is only transient. Sooner or later, you will be hit by bad news. If you are prepared for it, when bad news hits you, you won't feel that bad. You will just move on, as you are secure in the knowledge that all bad news has to be eventually followed by good news. This cycle is the nature of life.

The World of Duality

We live in a world of duality—pain and pleasure, hot and cold, up and down, positive and negative, happy and sad, good and bad, and so on. *Life is like a roller coaster ride. There will be ups and downs. The moment you realize this fact and develop a neutral attitude to both ups and downs in life, you become free.* You no longer depend on the next good news in life to make you feel happy nor do you let the next wave of bad news hit you hard. You remain naturally happy no matter what. This is a wonderful state to anchor yourself strongly to, and you will be able to do so if you practice even-mindedness daily.

Life Has No Animosity Toward You

"But," you may ask, "how do I do that?" You must start by recognizing that life has no animosity toward you. It's just carrying out its duty as you are carrying out your duties. It just happens that some life events are not what we expect, or what we like. For example, if an earthquake hits you, it has no personal animosity toward you. When a strong ocean wave thrashes your life boat, it doesn't have any animosity toward you. It's just its nature to do so. A whale is not affected by the huge waves in the ocean, right? It enjoys those waves and rides over them. What is bad for you is actually not bad for the whale, right? So, it is all a matter of relativity. *All events of life and all news are relative. What is good news for you could be bad news for others and vice versa.*

Then what is good and what is bad? Where is the truth? What is right?

We Live in a World of Separate Realities

It's very hard to pinpoint truth in this crazy world. We live in a world of separate realities. There are few absolute realities, such as the Earth is round and revolves around the Sun. Even that absolute truth was not evident to people, our ancestors, until the 15th century. An important point to realize here is that *our understanding of truth changes over time.* So, I say that there is no way for us to say whether Mr. Trump is either right or wrong. We just don't know. We think he is right or wrong based on our own perspectives and experiences in life at this moment. But, a year from now we may have a different perspective. Maybe 10 years from now everyone may say, "isn't it the best thing that Trump became our president?" That might sound radical, but you never know! *So, the point here is that if all we have is our perspective and we do not know the absolute truth, why worry and suffer?* Why instigate others or be instigated by others? Why act in haste? Why don't we simply say, "Let us respect each other's perspectives. Let us get along well with good faith and we will see what future holds for us." That's a refined way of conducting ourselves and our forefathers will be proud of us.

Express Yourself Freely but with Kindness

This doesn't mean you shouldn't exercise your individual rights of free speech and free expression of thoughts. You are free to express yourself but do so with kindness and with a lack of hatred in your heart. *Hatred, anger, and resentment burn you up more rapidly than the person you are projecting those negative emotions on to.* Anything can be said in this world when it is said with kindness and love. The hatred I see across the nation really bothers me. Aren't we civilized? Aren't we one of the most advanced nations on Earth? Aren't we supposed to lead others by example? Then why do we act and say things that are out of alignment with our true north principles?

Be Optimistic but Not to the Point of Foolishness

If you are a liberal, some of the first questions you might pose are, "Isn't Mr. Trump supposed to lead us by example? Why is he making such inflammatory statements, and why has he done what he has done in the past?" Those are legitimate questions. Unfortunately, we are not going to find answers to those questions, nor is it useful to steer yourself in that direction. The reason is this: Mr. Trump is what he is just as you are who you are, and I am who I am. *It's very hard to change the core of a being. That's an evolutionary process.* He is going to behave the way he is used to behaving for the past 70 years. Thinking that he is going to change at this late stage of his life is optimistic to the point of foolishness. If all the negative news and terrible mudslinging that occurred over the past year have not changed his ways, then he is not going to change now when he is in power. So, accept him for what he is and move on. That will save you a lot of suffering. Determine how you can align yourself with his government and do good for yourself and others. That's the best you can do. Really, that's the only answer that is viable.

Understand the Nature of the Person

A lion hunts, kills, and devours the flesh; a cow grazes, eats grass, and gives you milk; a butterfly drinks the nectar from the flowers, floats in the air, and is such a delight to watch. These are the natures of these creatures. You can't ask the lion to drink nectar or the cow to eat meat. It just doesn't work that way. You have to accept their nature and move on. That also applies to Trump. He is who he is. Many people tried to change him, including his own campaign managers, but they couldn't.

So, it's wise to move on. You may encounter incidences where Mr. Trump may say things or do things that are going to bother you. Or maybe he acts completely presidential. But, remember, if Mr. Trump says something that's not nice or acts in a way that's not decent, you don't have to reciprocate it. That's not you, and you don't need to try to be something that's not you. It is better to lead by example. Work on things you have control over and keep expanding your influence. You can do this no matter what's going on around you. Recall that when Marco Rubio, Jeb Bush, and others tried to imitate Trump by making harsh comments and saying negative things, it backfired on them. That's because it was not their nature. It just didn't fit them and ultimately led to their demise.

Be Good-Natured, and You Will Be Rewarded in the End

The people who survived this election campaign and came out

unscathed are honorable people like Dr. Ben Carson who refused to get into the mudslinging business no matter what was thrown at him or how unfairly he was treated. Everyone loved him on both sides of the aisle. He is a true gentleman and has followed the path of Christ and other great ones. He has forgiven all people who have done wrong to him and refused to harm them in return and, thus, has set a great example to follow.

Do you know why he was able to do that? Because he was even-minded. He was able to take all the news equally, whether he won or lost, whether he was treated fairly or unfairly, whether he got what he wanted or not. He did his best, under the given circumstances, and accepted whatever results he got. That's a very high state of living. It takes more courage, faith, and greatness to do this than to win. I know that he will be rewarded at the highest level by God.

I am reminded of a wonderful poem written on the wall of Mother Teresa's home, a beautiful poem that is a perfect example of even-mindedness:

People are often unreasonable, irrational, and self-centered.
Forgive them anyway.

If you are kind, people may accuse you of selfish, ulterior motives.
Be kind anyway.

If you are successful, you will win some
unfaithful friends and some genuine enemies.
Succeed anyway.

If you are honest and sincere people may deceive you.
Be honest and sincere anyway.
What you spend years creating, others could destroy overnight.
Create anyway.

If you find serenity and happiness, some may be jealous.
Be happy anyway.

The good you do today, will often be forgotten.
Do good anyway.

Give the best you have, and it will never be enough.
Give your best anyway.

In the final analysis, it is between you and God.
It was never between you and them anyway.

—Mother Teresa

 Dr. Calm's Recommended Exercises

1. The next time you are hit by a news you don't like, instead of reacting immediately, take a moment and think, "Is it a bad news? If so, is it bad news for me or bad news for all? If it's just a bad news for me and a

good news for others, then what is the real news? Isn't the real news always neutral, but we see it as either bad or good, depending on our perspective? If it is a bad news for a lot of people, then is it worth to react and act in a negative way? What is it going to do to my peace of mind? Can I choose to act gracefully?"

2. The next time you are hit by a news you don't like, avoid dwelling on it. If you are watching TV, stop watching. If you are reading a newspaper, stop reading. If you are in surroundings that propagate negativity, get away. Do not let the news persist and penetrate your peace of mind. Remind yourself that all good has to be followed by bad and all bad has to be followed by good. That's the nature of life.

3. The next time you see a potential conflict with a friend, family member, or colleague, stop for a moment and ask yourself, "Isn't everything in life is just a perspective, except for a few absolute truths? Whatever that I am saying or the other person is saying, isn't it just a perspective? Don't we all remain in our own unique personal worlds, creating our own personal realities? Then, why quarrel?"

Key No. 7
Empty Your Mind Before You Go to Sleep

Last but Not Least, Sleep Well

You may say, "How can I sleep well when the whole world is going crazy around me? How can I sleep well when every day there is some kind of bad news? As soon as I turn on the TV or read a newspaper, I am bombarded with negative information."

I understand that it's not easy, but there are solutions. *The first thing to do is to avoid being drawn into media sensationalism.*

Recently, I was talking to a magazine editor, and he said, "Unfortunately, the truth about major media outlets these days is that they love to publish sensational news whether it helps their audience or not, whether it is good or bad, whether it is true or false. Truth doesn't matter to them. Sensation creates an urge for people to buy into the news cycle and increase their viewership and circulation. That improves their revenue and helps them meet their financial bottom-line. So, that's what they do."

Be Wise. Avoid Being Drawn into the Media Sensationalism

Media sensationalism never ends. I thought it would end after the election was over. But it did not end. It continues with greater vigor now. The point is that media thrives on this. *Use your discretion when watching news. Choose your channels wisely.* One of my colleagues recently said, *"If you don't watch the news, you are uninformed. If you watch the news, you are misinformed."* That's so true. It is hard to remain not misinformed these days. The best thing to do is mind your own business. You don't need to watch all the news in this world.

Focus on What's Important in Life

You only have 24 hours a day, and you already have so much to do. Why burden yourself with negative news? The world is not going to stop functioning if you stop watching news. Keep it to a minimum. In particular, avoid watching or reading news for 2 to 3 hours before going to sleep. *All the information you absorb will overstimulate your brain, haunt you through the night, and prevent you from having a sound and peaceful sleep.* When you wake up in the morning, you can always catch up with the news if you want to.

Empty Your Mind Before Going to Sleep

A good way to empty our mind is by practicing the relaxation exercise and the meditation technique you learned earlier in this book. These help relax your mind, stop the restlessness, and instill calmness. *When your mind is calm and undisturbed, you will automatically have a sound sleep.*

Later in the day, avoid beverages that could stimulate your brain, like caffeine, tea, and high-energy drinks. Do not fall for addictions like smoking, alcohol, or drugs. They may give a feeling of temporary elation or sedation, but they mask the problem that is causing stress. In the long term, they are very damaging.

Make Sleep a Priority

No matter how busy you are or how much work you have to do, ensure that you get 6 to 8 hours of sleep. Sleep charges your body and mind battery. Can you imagine going to work during the day without charging your phone the night before? Your phone will stop performing and eventually will die on you. The same is true if you don't recharge your mind and body every night with sound and peaceful sleep; you won't be able to perform well during the day. You will be irritable, distracted, and error-prone. In the long term, people with chronic insomnia are at increased risk of experiencing heart attacks, high blood pressure, cancer, and ultimately death.

Do you know why most people can't sleep well even when they want to? It's because their minds are very restless with all the events and thoughts of the day. They just don't know how to shut down their mind. When they go to sleep, they carry those thoughts with them and thus have a disturbed sleep. During the day, they feel tired and sleepy and lack energy. The real solution for good sleep is to arrest restlessness and find calmness. When you practice calmness using the Laws of Thought Mechanics, relaxation exercises, and meditation techniques, you will automatically sleep well.

 Dr. Calm's Recommended Exercises

1. Every night, before going to sleep, practice the relaxation exercise and meditation technique given in this book. Even if you could do them for a few minutes sincerely, it will greatly improve the quality of your sleep.

2. If you find yourself having trouble sleeping at night, sometimes changing the place where you sleep helps. Or changing your sleep environment. Make it spa-like if you have to. Give importance to sleep. Prioritize it. Whatever we prioritize in life, we tend to find a way to make it happen.

Conclusion
Healing Post-Election Stress Disorder

It's about time that we the people come together as a nation and heal ourselves from the wounds sustained during one of the fiercest political battles of all time. Whether you are a conservative or a liberal; whether you are a democrat, a republican, or an independent; whether you are a Trump supporter or Clinton supporter; whether you are a Californian or Texan—it doesn't matter who you are, it's important that you heal, and you let other people around you heal. We all are human beings first, and then we have our affiliations to various parties and groups. We all are good people, and we all want to experience good in life. It's time that we let go of all the differences and come together as a nation.

I know it's hard. I know it's unexpected. I know for some people this is the worst nightmare of their lives. However, I also know that deep inside you are resilient and that peace of mind is your true nature. No matter what challenges are thrown at you, you have the ability to face them gracefully and emerge stronger and wiser. *When you face difficulties and feel like your happiness is lost,*

remember that the happiness you lost is the conditional happiness.
Your unconditional happiness is untouched and is waiting for you
beneath all the superficial tumults of life.

Your innate health is like the deep, peaceful ocean that remains
unperturbed despite the ferocious nature of the waves at the
surface. *Deep within you is a sacred place of peace untouched by
the chaos around you.* As long as you remember your true nature
and remain in touch with it, you will be alright.

As you understand the Laws of Thought Mechanics, you will
understand that *all thoughts are transient and only create a
momentary reality.* Whatever you are thinking at this time feels
real to you, but once those thoughts pass and are replaced by
other thoughts, your reality changes. When negative thoughts
enter your mind, ignore them. If you do so, the next positive
thought waiting in line comes forward and washes the negative
ones away. That is how you remain in a naturally peaceful and
happy state of mind. Do not pay too much attention to negative
thoughts. The more attention you pay to them, the worse you are
going to feel.

*Sometimes, as much as you know that you should ignore negative
thoughts, it is not always easy.* The relaxation exercise described
earlier will help you let go of them. All you need to do is
practice it for 5 to 10 minutes. You will feel the difference. You
can practice this exercise as many times as you want during
the day and whenever you need it. It's like a powerful tool at
your disposal. *To delve into the depths of calmness, meditation
is necessary.* The meditation technique provided is time tested

and, when practiced sincerely and daily, will help you reap great benefits.

Avoid quarrels with people, especially your loved ones, family members, friends, and colleagues. They have their opinions about the election and Mr. Trump just as you do. Respect them. You can agree to disagree. Recently, I witnessed a mother not allowing her 10-year-old child back home because he supported Trump at school. The grandmother of one of my colleagues wouldn't allow her grandchild to visit for Christmas because the 19-year-old grandson supported Trump. This is terrible! I have seen friends of my friends get into arguments at Starbucks, restaurants, and other public places. I have seen relationships broken, friends separated, and other bad outcomes as a result of these arguments. So, avoid them by all means. Don't say unkind things to people around you, lest you regret it later. Remain cool-headed. Move on, march forward, and never look back!

Bonus Key
No Situation Is Absolutely Hopeless

The Four Forces that Propel You Out of Despair

There will be times in your life—no matter what you do and how hard you try— when life's challenges will cause extreme misery and sorrow. It is as if all your efforts are in vain. You feel as if you are stuck in a tunnel of despair. Everything around you looks dark and uncertain. It seems like things are falling apart and your world is coming to an end. It's very hard to see a way out of your problems when you are stuck in the tunnel of despair. During these times, there are four essential thought forces that can help lead you out of this dark tunnel.

Hope

First, there is hope. Without hope, nothing moves forward in life. People can do terrible things to themselves and others when they feel hopeless. They might commit suicide or even think about killing others. So the most important thing you have to develop is the power of hope. You should never say your situation is hopeless; to say that your situation is hopeless means to doubt the infinite power you have within you.

This Universe is not designed to be scarce. The default design of this Universe is abundance. Our Universe is designed to provide for all the needs of the trillions of living beings in this world with abundance. Those who find strength to see at least a ray of hope, even in the darkest hours of their lives, will definitely find a way out of their problems. This is an inescapable truth of life. It is the power of hope that helps people see the light at the end of the tunnel. The stronger the feeling of hope, the easier it is to emerge out of the tunnel of despair.

Faith

But hope alone is not sufficient to emerge out of the tunnel of despair. While you see the light at the end of the tunnel, you also need to make an effort to emerge from it. As you travel through this dark tunnel of despair, your abilities will be tested and doubt will arise in your mind. The beginning of doubt in your mind means the beginning of the erosion of your self-confidence. But during those times of self-doubt, it is the power of faith that propels you forward. Deep inside, if you have faith that things will get better no matter how difficult your situation is today, it will help you overcome your self-doubt. Know that this Universe is designed not to fill you with doubt and despair, although for a superficial thinker it might seem so. Life tests and challenges you to ignite your willpower so that you might awaken your innate and infinite abilities to overcome these challenges and move closer and closer toward perfection. And with this power of faith, you will move forward swiftly in life.

Patience

As you propel yourself forward through this tunnel of despair, with faith and hope, you still might not find the solutions that you are looking for. Sometimes, it seems as if there is no end to this tunnel. To emerge successfully, along with faith and hope, you also need patience. Be patient until you reach the other end of the tunnel where it is full of light, where you see everything clearly and find what you want in life. You just can't say, "I am hopeful and have faith and I need solutions right away. I can't wait!" Well, sometimes you might get your answers immediately but not always. Patience is a virtue. Those people who do not have enough patience will lose in their lives despite any other great capabilities they have. So keep trying and stay patient. If you do so, it is absolutely certain that you will emerge victorious from any difficult and dark situation in your life.

Endurance

As you move forward with patience, your endurance will be tested. Obstacles might arise in your path. With every obstacle, make sure that your resolve gets stronger to win and not weaker. Life is not a sprint; it is a marathon. To run a sprint, a short burst of energy is sufficient. But to run a marathon, you need to maintain sustained levels of energy and endurance. The only way to develop this endurance is to keep trying and pushing yourself forward tirelessly through all obstacles. One day, you will develop so much endurance that you will finally run the marathon of your life with ease. Although everyone and everything around you is falling apart, you will remain strong and unshakable. Imagine yourself having that invincible power of an absolutely calm state of mind. Such a feeling is very uplifting and will provide you with energy and endurance to move forward despite all obstacles in your path. You finally emerge from the tunnel of despair, penetrating the darkness around you. Bathed in that revealing, brilliant light at the end of the tunnel, you feel relieved, refreshed, and rejuvenated.

The following experience from my life demonstrates the power of the four forces we discussed above.

At one time in my life, I was in deep distress and felt like my life was about to fall apart. There was a major conflict between two of my very close family members and I was caught in the middle. I felt that the emotional pain and suffering during that stage of my life was enormous. Both family members were important to me, and for the prosperity of my family, I couldn't see either one of them hurt or unhappy. I tried everything I could, but I could not find a solution to bring them together again. I thought, "What's going on? I am the stress management expert, and I can't even keep my own family happy and stress-free?"

Thoughts of despair, anger, frustration, and fear surrounded me. I felt stuck in my life. I did not see a bright future. It was during those extremely tough times that I discovered these four forces of hope, faith, patience, and endurance, which helped me to successfully and happily emerge from the tunnel of despair and find a win–win solution for all. Remember, sometimes even though you know that you are doing the right thing and you are applying all the right principles, life still has its own time line and way of sorting things out. Be patient. When the time is right, things will settle down by themselves. Meanwhile, it is important to stick to the right path and not be impulsive and impatient.

During that time, I was feeling very impulsive and I could have easily said nasty things to the others around me, which would have further jeopardized the relationships. "But," I asked myself, "is it the right thing to do? Should I say nasty things impulsively?" The answer from my conscience was very clear. Do not do it! So, I didn't, and I am glad that I didn't. After enduring the situation for more than three weeks, with continuous, open communication, affirming the love and affection that I have toward each of my family members, I was able to connect everyone together again. Everyone was happy. Everyone learned from their mistakes, all the negative energy was sucked away, and positive feelings were restored.

Remember, there is always light at the end of the tunnel. As you get closer and closer to that end, the presence of that light will be more and more evident. Just make the effort to go all the way through the tunnel!

Dr. Calm's Recommendations

1. The most important thing we all have to develop is the power of hope. We should never say our situation is hopeless.

2. This Universe is not designed to be scarce. The default design of this Universe is abundance.

3. The stronger the hope, the easier it is to emerge from the tunnel of despair.

4. The beginning of doubt in your mind means the beginning of erosion of your self-confidence. But during those times of self-doubt, it is the power of faith that propels you forward.

5. To successfully emerge from difficult situations of life, along with faith and hope, you also need patience. It is absolutely certain that you will emerge victorious from any dark situation in your life if you practice patience.

6. With every obstacle in your path to success, make sure that your resolve gets stronger to win, and not weaker.

7. Life is not a sprint; it is a marathon. To run a marathon, you need to maintain sustained levels of energy and develop endurance.

Bonus Key
How to Overcome Mood Swings

Moods—The Greatest Enemy to Your Relationships

So many people in this world are victims of mood swings. One moment they are fine, and the next moment, heaven only knows why, they turn moody. Moodiness is not good. It makes you quite unpredictable, and people around you might start avoiding you if you are always moody. By being irritable, you not only create misery for yourself but also for your family and friends. Just because people continue to tolerate you and your moods, it does not give you permission to continue to be temperamental. One day, even the most patient and kindhearted person who has silently tolerated your moods for years might leave you because over time, a bad temper can erode other people's good feelings for you. This is especially true in a close relationship like marriage where one person's moods and behavior strongly affect the partner. So, get a handle on your emotions and stop being moody today!

What Makes You Moody?

People often wonder what makes them moody. It is your
bad habits of thinking that cause moodiness. Knowingly
or unknowingly, some people carry these tendencies from
childhood, and over time, they turn into strong habits. Children
might learn these traits from their parents and other adults
whom they observe. If children are not taught early how to
correctly handle their emotions and their moods, they develop
maladaptive behaviors. It is important to teach your children how
their thoughts determine their emotions and moods, and how
they can choose good and positive ones.

Good Moods vs. Bad Moods

In your mind, thoughts flow freely. As long as you let them flow
freely, you remain happy and peaceful. That is a good mood.
The moment you block the flow of thoughts in your mind by
attaching to thoughts, you impede their natural flow and you feel
unhappy and distressed. That's a bad mood.

Although I stated this in the previous chapter and elsewhere, it
bears repeating here in this context. As thoughts flow in your
mind, you tend to get attached to past negative experiences or an
imagined, fearful future. Persistent focus on such thoughts leads
to a bad mood, and soon you find yourself worrying. The way to
reclaim your emotional health and maintain a good mood is to
let go of the unwholesome thoughts in your mind by practicing
thought detachment by saying, "It doesn't matter. It is just a
thought." Surely, they will flee.

Why Do People Overreact?

Some people overreact to every little thing. That's because they are in a bad mood. Moods often determine your response to stressors. Do you remember a day in your life when you were so stressed and everything that happened around you became irritating? There are days when you go to work and try to carry on with your job, but either because your boss reprimanded you that morning or you have a big bill to pay in the next few days or your kid is sick at home waiting for you or because of something else, you are so stressed that everything around you starts annoying you. Even usually innocuous sounds can elicit a bad response from you—the ringing phone, the chiming text message, the swooshing e-mail—everything becomes a source of irritation. However, the truth is that they are not to blame. It's your own bad mood that attracts like a magnet the sharp nails of stressors that turn your day into a painful series of adverse events.

Sometimes, we are emotionally sensitive and overreact in a similar way to being physically sensitive, as illustrated by the following real-life example.

One of my friends related this story to me.

A few years ago, I had some back pain and went for physical therapy. When the therapist started applying pressure to my back, there were certain places on my back that were very painful, and some places that were not. Wincing in pain, I retorted, "Why do you apply so much pressure on certain parts and less pressure on others? It's really painful."

The therapist courteously replied, "Sir! I have been applying the same pressure all over your back, but it seems that there are certain sore spots on your back that are causing pain even with minimal pressure."

I thought, "All this time I am blaming the therapist for applying too much pressure on my back, but in fact, it's my internal sore spots that are causing the pain and not the external pressure being applied."

Isn't it the same way with regard to our emotional reactivity? There are certain people who are emotionally very sensitive, and it does not take much to elicit a bad response from them. It seems that they have emotional sore spots in their minds that can be easily triggered even by minor pressures of life.

A Good Mood Is a Cushion of Invincibility

However, when you are in a good mood, you develop a cushion of protection around you, and these nails of stressors cannot penetrate your calm and happy state of mind. When you are in a good mood, even when bad things happen around you, you take them in stride and move on. You easily see solutions to your problems and effortlessly overcome them. You finish the tasks at hand efficiently and enjoy the free time you have earned as a result. Moreover, you are emotionally strong. You remain poised even under the enormous pressures of life's challenges. You stand unshaken even in the midst of worlds falling apart. You remain calm in the midst of chaos.

Good Mood and Stress Can't Live Together
Even-Mindedness Is the Solution to Moodiness

If you try to keep yourself in a good mood, stress walks out of
your life. A good mood and stress can't live together. Fake it
until you make it! When you feel distressed from inside, don't
let it overflow to the outside. Keep smiling and be composed.
I am not advising you not to address the challenges you face. I
am just saying keep calm and don't yield to moods, even under
pressure. With practice, you will be able to win over your moods.
Eventually, you will be transformed from a moody person into an
emotionally stable person.

How to Put Yourself in a Good Mood

There are three simple ways to put yourself in a good mood:

1. Let your thoughts flow freely in your mind. It's natural
   for thoughts to flow effortlessly in your mind. As long
   as you do not obstruct them, you will be fine. Good
   moods will follow you automatically. It is as simple as
   that.

2. Do not pay attention to negative thoughts, even
   though you may feel compelled to do so. If you already
   find yourself in a bad mood because you focused on
   negative thoughts, turn your attention away from
   them. Just do not yield to them. The moment you
   decide to turn away from them, the natural flow of

positive thoughts will wash them away and you will find yourself in a good mood again.

3. Focus on happy thoughts. Whatever thoughts you choose to focus become your moods. Focus on happy thoughts and you will find yourself in a happy mood. Focus on sad thoughts and I guarantee that you will find yourself in a bad mood. It is as easy as that. Know that you have the power to choose what thoughts you want to focus on and how you want to feel. Even though you are facing difficult circumstances, see beyond them and focus on something positive. The truth of life is that even in those situations where everything looks hopeless, you can always find a ray of hope and positivity in life. If necessary, create happy thoughts. That's also under your control!

Be the Hero of Your Life

If you keep smiling inwardly and maintain an attitude of even-mindedness at all times, external circumstances will affect you less. Your own internal world will rule your life. Anyone can smile when things are going well in their life. But only a hero can smile even when things are not going well. A hero knows every difficulty in life is a temporary phase, and sooner or later, that tough phase in life has to pass and a good phase must arrive. A hero knows that's the nature of life. Decide today that is the way you want to live the rest of your life. Be the hero of your life!

Dr. Calm's Recommendations

1. Moodiness results in unpredictable emotions and actions, thus making it very difficult for people around you to understand and get along with you. They will live in a constant state of doubt and fear not knowing what will set you off in the wrong direction.

2. No one likes to stay around moody people, especially in close relationships. Your moodiness can adversely affect the relationship. Take control of your moods today before it is too late.

3. Moodiness results from bad habits of thinking that get solidified into moods over time. The seeds for moodiness are often sowed in your childhood. But you can undo them by conscious choice.

4. By developing the habit of calmness and learning how to put yourself in a good mood at will, you become invincible to mood swings.

5. Next time, when a negative mood approaches you, watch and laugh at it. Tell the mood that you are awake. You are present. In that state of wakefulness, moods cannot bother you. As you practice this daily,

eventually all the bad moods relinquish their grip on you.

6. It is essential to put yourself in a good mood consistently for maximal success in life. When you are in good mood, it is much easier to accomplish the tasks at hand and much easier to find solutions to your problems.

7. The secret to putting yourself in a good mood is to (1) let your thoughts flow freely in your mind, (2) not focus on negative thoughts, and (3) direct your mind to focus on positive thoughts.

Peace of Mind in a Nutshell

Never Lose Hope

- The world is not coming to an end.

- Many unexpected things have happened in the history of this world. A majority of the world still survived them, right? So, we will survive this also

Move On, March Forward, and Never Look Back

- Now that the election is over, move on swiftly with your job, business, or other activities. At the end of the day, that is what is important.

- The conscious choices you make every day in your life will determine your destiny more than the election result. You control your destiny.

Realize That Every Thing Happens for a Reason

- It's time to get over the election results. Of course, you fought well and did the best you could for your candidate.

- Life is not perfect. You don't always get what you want. That's the harsh truth of life.

- When you accept this fact, life becomes more enjoyable.

Stay Away from Quarrels

- Do not argue with your friends, colleagues, and other people around you and cause yourself stress.

- When you argue and say unkind things to people around you, you will regret it later.

Realize That Failure Is the Stepping Stone for Success

- To expect not to fail in life is naive. To not to get up after falling down is stupid.

- So arise, awaken, and march forward. The next big thing in your life is waiting for you.

- "The season of failure is the best time for sowing the seeds of success." – Paramahansa Yogananda

- Come to an acceptance of the situation, and use this opportunity to transform your life.

Get Up Every Time You Fall

- The single most important quality that helps you succeed despite debacles in life is your ability to get up and move on.

- It's not how many times you fall but how many times you rise after each fall that determines your destiny.

Do Not Dwell on the Past; Worrying About the Past Doesn't Help

- The past has no life of its own. It is just a memory that exists in your mind and bothers you only to the extent you think about it.

- The more you ruminate over the past hurt, the worse you feel. So do not ruminate over the election results. It will lose its grip on you if you decide not to ruminate over it.

Letting Go Is the Only Solution

- Holding on to past hurt is like holding on to hot coal in your hand. It's going to burn you to pain. So, just let go.

- Letting go and embracing the future is the only way to get over the bitter feelings of this election.

- When you let go of the old thoughts, new thoughts will have the chance to flourish and bring good feelings to your life.

Never Imagine a Fearful Future; Realize That Future Is Just a Figment of Your Imagination

- Your inquiry into the future can be endless and it is often fear-driven. Don't fall into that trap.

- The fearful future is not real and is not yet here. Then why imagine a terrible future? Maybe everything will turn out good.

- The future holds promise if you let go of the past. Learn from the past, stay in the present, and plan for the future.

Anchor Yourself to the Present

- Living in the present moment eliminates stress from your life. Know that there is only one moment—this moment.

- The next moment has not come yet. What ever happened a moment ago is no longer present. So just live in the moment.

Stay Calm

- Stress can lead to major health problems like heart attacks, strokes, accidents, and worse, but practicing calmness will protect you.

- When you are calm, your mind becomes clear and reveals solutions that you never thought about before.

Exercise Your Conscious Will and Avoid Being Drawn into the Media Sensationalism

- The media may project news as if the world is falling apart and is coming to an end. It's their job to do so to make the news sensational. That improves their viewership and thus their revenue.

- Don't fall for the media sensationalism. Guard yourself against the barrage of negative news attacks. The more you focus on the negative information, the worse you are going to feel.

Divert Your Mind to Something You Enjoy

- Know that your mind feels whatever you feed it.

- Watch your favorite movie, go for a walk, listen to music, read a book, play a game, or do an activity you enjoy that distracts you from the news cycle.

Practice Even-Mindedness

- Learn to take any and all news with even-mindedness. The key to protecting your peace of mind after this crazy election cycle is to practice even-mindedness.

- Even-mindedness means viewing all news and information with a sense of calm, with a sense of total acceptance.

- Practice saying, "I don't mind whatever happens." This will help you remain unruffled no matter what unfolds in the next few years.

Empty Your Mind Before You Go to Sleep

- The news events of the day overstimulate your brain, haunt you through the night, and steal your peaceful sleep.
- Stop watching or reading news 2 to 3 hours before going to bed. This will help your mind relax.
- When you wake up in the morning, you can catch up with the news if you want to.

Other Products by the Author

Books (coming soon)

- *Calm in the Midst of Chaos: A Busy but Happy Doctor's Prescription for Stress-Free Living*

Audio and DVD (coming soon)

- Your Personal Stress Reduction Program: Live Longer Live Younger. *Better Health through Stress-Mastery.*

- Stress Mastery for Health Professionals: Reignite Your Passion and Reinvent Your Life. *Every Day You Save So Many Lives. Don't Forget to Save Your Own!*

- Corporate Stress-Reduction Program: Stress Minimum Performance Maximum. *How to Defeat Stress and Skyrocket Your Company's Performance.*

Speaking Presentations Keynote

- Exclusively designed and refined to create the ***most powerful*** *impact in the least amount of time*, Dr. Kiran Dintyala's signature keynote presentation takes the audience through a stunning set of illustrations and slides.

- Combined with his *calming presence*, this 40-minute presentation invokes deep peace, joy, and meaningful insights that are life-changing.

Just sit back, relax, and watch the show. You are sure to be thrilled!

At the end of the presentation, you will be able to ask Dr. Kiran Dintyala the questions you want and *get personal attention*. Book Dr. Kiran Dintyala now for a keynote presentation at your organization.

Half to Full-day Seminars

- Explore the PET system for stress-free living in depth. Transform your life forever with this *calming and insightful* interaction with Dr. Dintyala.

- You will be able to question, discuss, and understand a wide range of topics from *acute stress vs. chronic stress* to internal vs. external sources of stress to the **true vs. false sources of stress in your life.**

- As you uncover these concepts, a natural and simple understanding of the *true source of stress in your life* will be revealed to you. This fascinating new understanding will wisely guide you to the long-sought shores of happiness and success in life.

You will feel a sense of freedom from all worries, fear, and anxiety in your life. You will finally be able to learn how to *let go of any negative emotions harbored in your heart.*

Ultimately, *a natural peace, joy, and contentment will fill your being from within*—your life will be completely transformed. Don't miss it!!!

Weekend or Weeklong Retreats

Don't you want to *get away* once in a while from all worldly obligations and *just relax*? Life in our modern society can be burdening you to the point of exhaustion, crushing you under the weight of all your responsibilities and endless hard work.

I used to ask myself, *how can we prevent stress? How can we remain calm and joyful even under challenging circumstances? How do we sustain that energy and joy even after we come back from a vacation?* The answer lies in the question itself. What do we do when we get away? Of course, we chillax and enjoy, but do we learn or do anything new that's going to sustain our joy even after we return from a vacation?

For most people, the answer is "no"! In fact, in our current world, *it's so hard to take our eyes off the electronic gadgets*, and most people end up bringing their work responsibilities on vacation, too! This leaves their spouses and other family members irritated and unhappy, leading to more stress. Some people have a good time with their families, do a lot of fun activities, and truly relax—which is excellent. But, when they get back to work, again, they fall into the old ways, which leads to stress again.

The solution for this problem is **not only to enjoy your vacation but also learn something new and exciting** that will help you get back to your daily activities with more passion and sustain your peace, joy, and balance as you carry out your daily activities.

At this retreat, you will meet **the foremost experts** in this field who will guide you to **find peace, joy, wisdom**, and much more. You will learn some of the **simplest yet most beneficial exercises for your health**, and we will do them along with you as guides.

We will practice **relaxation techniques** together, and I will personally train you to master these techniques. All these things will result in **an ultimate experience of peace, joy, and balance in life.** The most important thing is that you will be able to **sustain that experience even after you leave** the retreat.

This is the **"Ultimate Truth Finding Program"** that gives you the ultimate freedom, peace, joy, and balance in your life. Don't wait anymore. Let's get together and experience the ultimate peace, joy, and wisdom together!

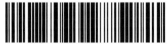

Made in the USA
San Bernardino, CA
03 February 2017